WHEN MEMORY FADES AWAY

Autor: Jorge Javier Bergues Mustelier

Dedication

To my family, for being my refuge in every storm, for the unconditional love and shared strength you have given me throughout this journey. You are the driving force that keeps me moving forward, always.

To my teachers, who not only taught me knowledge but also how to question, to always seek the truth, and to find value in continuous learning. Thank you for guiding me with wisdom and patience every step of the way.

To my friends, for standing by my side in moments of light and shadow, for every word of encouragement, every shared laugh, and every silence that spoke volumes. You are my network, my chosen family.

And to my patients, who teach me daily the true meaning of struggle, resilience, and hope. This book is for you, because in each of your stories I find the inspiration to continue, to learn, and to do everything possible to walk alongside you on the path to a better life.

This book is for all of you.

Prologue: A Journey Through Forgetfulness

Imagine waking up one day and not remembering the names of the people you love. It's not just a simple lapse; it's a dense fog that envelops your mind, erasing important moments and blurring the lines of your own story. This is Clara's reality, a woman trapped in a body and mind that are slowly fading, as Alzheimer's and diabetes conspire to rob her of the most precious thing she has: her memory, her essence.

But this is not just Clara's story. It is also Leticia's story, her daughter, who faces the devastation of watching her mother gradually slip away. It reflects the experience of so many families who struggle in silence, witnessing how connections that once seemed unbreakable are shattered under the weight of unforgiving diseases. Facing Alzheimer's is not just a battle against forgetfulness; it is a battle for identity, for love, for life itself.

In my 20 years of experience as a physician, I have met many Claras and Leticias. It's a reality we live every day, and through this work, I aim to raise awareness, beyond just a talk about a disease that, to a large extent, can be prevented.

Throughout these pages, we will explore not only loss but also resilience, the legacy of love that transcends illness, and the importance of taking care of our present to safeguard our future. This novel is a mirror that invites us to reflect on our own lives, the memories we take for granted, and the fragility of the human mind.

With a modern language and a powerful narrative, *The Empty Reality* is not just a story about illness; it's a story of struggle, bravery, and hope. It reminds us that, while time may erase memories, the love we sow remains, even when everything else is lost.

Join Leticia and Clara on this journey filled with intense emotions, and discover how, despite the darkness, there is always a spark of light shining deep within the mind and heart.

This is a story that touches the core of our humanity. Are you ready to discover it?

Chapter 1: The Encroaching Forgetfulness

Doña Clara was sitting in her favorite armchair, the one that had accompanied every stage of her life. The upholstery, though somewhat worn, still retained the warm color of the days when her children played around her. From there, she had watched them grow, heard their laughter fill the house, and seen their arguments grow sharper as they ventured into adolescence. That chair was a silent witness to her story, a refuge where Clara would rest after long workdays, and where, in recent years, she had spent more and more time.

The sunlight streamed through the living room window, illuminating objects that had once held meaning. There were photographs on the walls, but Clara struggled to identify each face. She knew those people, those smiles, those eyes, belonged to someone important in her life, but she could no longer place the names or the stories that had once accompanied them. She looked at the photos as one might look at a landscape through a fogged window; the details slipped through the fingers of her mind.

There was a strange feeling, a shadow looming over her, but she couldn't explain it. It was as if something was hiding in the crevices of her mind, something that stole her clarity. Today, more than on other days, that mental fog felt thicker. She shifted slightly in the armchair with a soft sigh, her hands resting on her knees, fingers intertwined in a gesture that betrayed her confusion.

"What was it that I had to do?" she wondered. She knew there was something, but no matter how hard she tried, she couldn't remember what it was. She felt as if her memory, once a constant stream of thoughts, was slowly evaporating, as if the relentless sun of the years had dried it up without her realizing it. She tried to focus, to search in some corner of her brain for the answer that eluded her. What was it?

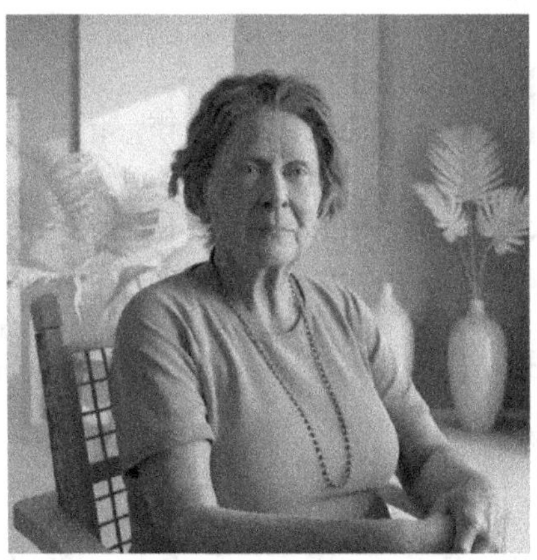

With effort, she stood up. Her movements were slow, and each step seemed like a small challenge. She walked toward the kitchen, hoping that by moving, her mind would clear and that the answers would appear in the least expected place, as they often did when she distracted herself. She opened a drawer with trembling hands and began searching without knowing exactly what she was looking for. Her breathing quickened. Desperation started to seep through the cracks of her apparent calm. The drawers filled with empty sounds, objects clattering against each other, but none of them brought her the answer.

"¿Clara, what are you doing?"

Leticia's voice pulled her out of the trance. Her daughter stood in the kitchen doorway, looking at her with that mixture of tenderness and concern that Clara knew so well. Leticia, the eldest of her children, had always been the one to bear the burden of caregiving. Though Clara never mentioned it, she could feel the weight that this unasked-for responsibility placed on her daughter.

"Looking for the keys again?" Leticia asked with a soft smile. "You left them on the table a little while ago."

Clara turned her head toward the table, and there they were—the keys—gleaming under the light streaming through the window. She walked toward them with slow steps, as if delaying the moment of confronting the truth that this scene revealed. She had forgotten. Again.

She looked at Leticia. A faint smile crossed her face, but behind that smile was confusion, and a latent fear that she dared not confess, even to herself. She didn't remember talking to Leticia that day, nor leaving the keys. The fact that Leticia seemed so sure of what had happened made her doubt her own reality even more. What else had she forgotten? What else had gotten lost in that fog invading her mind?

Leticia, with her typical worried-mother expression, approached and picked up the keys. "Mom, you've got to stop wandering around looking for things. You need to rest. Come, sit with me for a while," she said, guiding her back to the living room. Clara allowed herself to be led, though deep inside, she couldn't shake the feeling of loss—of something deeper than just the keys.

Conversations with Leticia were like flashes. Clara could remember fragments, isolated moments that, like pieces of a puzzle, seemed to fit together for brief moments but then faded as if they had never existed. Was this the first time they had talked about this? Had they had this conversation before? A part of Clara knew they had, that it wasn't the first time she had forgotten something important, but another, more confused part, couldn't be sure of anything.

"We've talked about this before, haven't we?" Clara asked, her voice trembling, hoping for a comforting answer but knowing it wouldn't come.

Leticia nodded gently, and in her eyes, Clara saw that look of concern she feared so much. That look that reminded her that things were not okay, that something in her mind was failing.

The clock on the wall gave a small click, marking the passing hours, as if each second ticking by was a countdown. Clara looked at the clock but couldn't remember if it was morning or afternoon. How long had it been since the last time she felt clarity? Was it yesterday or weeks ago? Months, perhaps? Everything was so blurry.

Leticia, sitting next to her on the couch, began talking about her day, trying to distract her, to pull her out of that loop of thoughts that threatened to consume her. Clara smiled and nodded at what seemed like the appropriate moments, but deep down, she knew she could barely follow the conversation. Her daughter's words were like echoes, reverberating in her mind without form or structure, dissipating before she could grasp them.

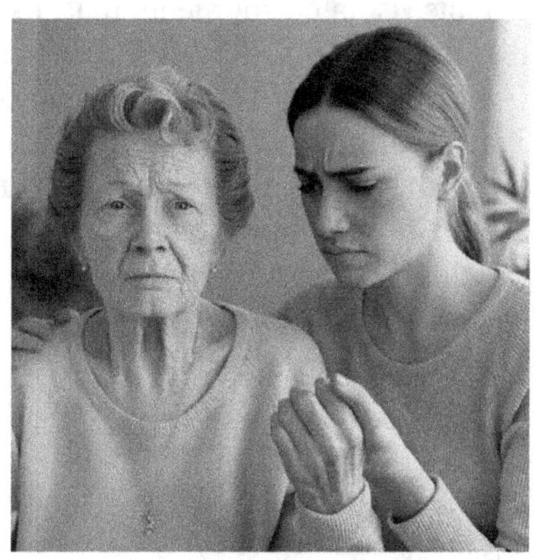

Leticia looked at her, waiting for a response. Clara opened her mouth to speak, but the words wouldn't come. She wasn't sure what she was supposed to say. Then, after a silence that seemed to stretch longer than usual, she let out a sigh. "I'm sorry, my dear, I'm so sorry..."

At that moment, Leticia took her hand, squeezing it tightly. "You don't have to apologize, Mom. I'm here with you. I'll always be here."

But Clara, though grateful, couldn't help feeling that, little by little, she was slipping away. She was drifting, like a ship gliding into the fog, moving further from the shore, unsure if she would ever find her way back.

Chapter 2: Inside the Mind

The scene shifts abruptly. We are no longer in Doña Clara's living room, where time seemed to pass along an imprecise line, wrapped in the fog of forgetfulness. Now, the space around her transforms into a vast internal landscape, a symbolic representation of her mind. We delve deep into her brain, a place that is no longer the vibrant and robust network of connections it once was, but rather a fraying fabric exposed to the winds of time.

The ground beneath our feet is not solid but a mixture of memories and sensations floating in the air like golden threads. These threads weave together the most important moments of her life: the first time she held her daughter Leticia in her arms, her wedding day, the laughter of her grandchildren running through the garden. These were once unbreakable threads, braided with the strength of life, but now they begin to lose their luster. In the distance, some of these threads unravel almost imperceptibly, as if they were strands of an old loom that can no longer hold its structure.

As we venture further into Clara's mind, the golden threads become scarce. We approach a darker area, where memories are no longer whole, and the connections between neurons weaken. Here, Alzheimer's leaves its mark. We see how neurons, once active and full of life, now seem fragile. Some simply shut down. The emptiness is palpable, an overwhelming silence where there was once activity and electrical sparks. The neuronal landscape is desolate: where there was once a dense network of vibrant connections, now only fragments remain, pieces of what was once a mind full of memories, experiences, and identity.

Fog covers much of this cerebral landscape, erasing the pathways between memories. The faces of her loved ones, once clear, begin to fade into the distance. Inside her own brain, Doña Clara searches desperately for those lost threads. She wants to remember. She knows there is something important, something she must hold on to, but the more she tries to grasp those threads, the faster they seem to disintegrate. It is a cruel game, one she cannot win.

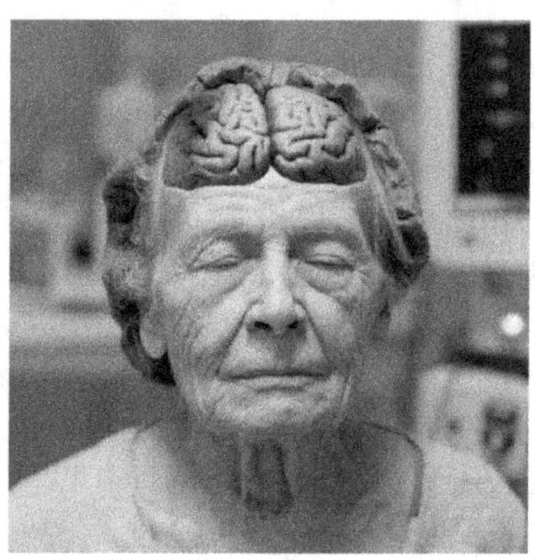

It's Alzheimer's, the relentless disease that not only steals memories but strips a person of their very essence. Doña Clara is neither the first nor the last to face this cruel fate, but within her mind, each loss feels like a small personal apocalypse. It's not simply forgetting a conversation—it's the loss of the connections that once defined her as a mother, wife, and friend.

The Sandcastles of Memory

As we continue exploring this internal representation of Clara's mind, a subtle but powerful shift brings us to a new realization: Alzheimer's is not the only enemy. There is another dark force working in the shadows, a silent enemy that has been eroding her mental connections without her even noticing. Diabetes.

Diabetes has been affecting her brain for years, slowly eroding her cells' ability to receive the energy they need. The neurons, which once thrived on glucose, now struggle to maintain balance. The connections between them crumble like sandcastles battered by the waves.

We can see how the nerve fibers, once strong and robust, are now weakened by insulin resistance. The brain cells, accustomed to a life of abundance, are now in a state of hunger. It's an internal battle Clara cannot even feel, but the impact is devastating. Each day, her brain loses its ability to function as it should. Every small lapse, every moment of confusion, is a reminder of this hidden battle.

In this mental theater, the connections that were once firm and solid are now falling apart. The memories of her grandchildren's laughter, her late husband's embraces, and the simple moments of daily joy are swept away by this relentless current. It's a constant struggle between two destructive forces, each in its own way dismantling what was once fertile ground for memories.

The Desolate Landscape

We now find ourselves in a space that was once colorful and vibrant but is now covered in shadows. Clara's mental landscape has become a desolate expanse, where the towers of memories that once stood proudly are collapsing one after another. In the distance, a few structures remain standing—the oldest memories, those that have resisted the passage of time. But even these are beginning to show signs of wear.

It is a mental landscape that resembles a battlefield after the storm. Fragments of memories are scattered everywhere; some still shine with a faint golden glow, but others are broken, irreparable. Clara tries to walk among them, as if she could gather the pieces and rebuild them, but she knows it's an impossible task.

The Imminent Presence of Forgetfulness

In this vast inner landscape, the sense of loss is constant. Doña Clara confronts her own mind, fighting to hold on to what she can still remember. However, the presence of forgetfulness is imminent. It feels like a shadow lurking in the deepest corners of her brain, an unstoppable force consuming everything.

Alzheimer's has advanced silently, and now its impact is visible in every corner of her mind. What was once a vibrant and lively place is now plagued with emptiness and darkness. The lights that once illuminated her memory are dimming one by one. Even the most basic memories, like her children's names or daily moments, are fading away.

But she is not alone. Alongside Alzheimer's, diabetes continues its destructive course, accelerating the deterioration, making the loss even quicker and more devastating. It's a macabre dance, a collaboration between two diseases that have taken control of her mind and are tearing it apart from within.

A Lost Battle

The journey through Clara's mind is a brutal reminder of what it means to lose memory, to lose oneself. It's not just a matter of forgetting a name or a place. It's much deeper. It's the unraveling of everything one is, of everything one has lived.

As we witness the collapse of her memories, we can't help but feel a deep sadness. Clara is not just a victim of her own mind; she is a victim of the biological forces conspiring against her, eroding her ability to remember, to feel, to be herself.

In this mental labyrinth, there is no way out. The neurons that once easily intertwined, creating memories and emotions, are now dying, one by one. And Clara, trapped in this dark place, is losing not only her memory but also her connection to everything she once loved.

Chapter 3: The Empty Reality

Clara holds the family photo with both hands, her fingers tracing the frame with an almost ritualistic gentleness, as if physical contact with that image could somehow restore what she has lost. Her fingertips caress the smiling faces that appear before her: three generations, all gathered, frozen in a moment of eternal happiness that now exists only in that picture. In the distance, a breeze enters through a partially open window, lightly lifting the curtains, but Clara doesn't notice. She is absorbed, trapped in a space between the present and a past that feels increasingly out of reach.

She knows the people in the photo are her family. She feels it deep within, in the most intimate corner of her heart, a place that has not yet been fully touched by the fog enveloping her mind. She doesn't need to remember the details to know that she once loved them intensely. But the faces in the photograph are starting to fade—not because of the quality of the paper or the passage of time, but due to something far more painful: her memory is erasing them.

She strokes the face of a man in the photo. He is her husband— or at least, he was. She knows this because a part of her remembers the warmth of his presence, the security she felt when he was by her side. But his name, their conversations, the moments they shared—all of that has been lost in the vast fog covering her mind. She looks at his smile, tries to recall the sound of his laughter, but she cannot. It's like trying to catch smoke with her hands.

Alzheimer's has done its work silently, stealing her memories one by one, like a thief operating in the dark, taking small pieces until what remains is a fragmented and empty version of her life. But Alzheimer's hasn't been working alone. Diabetes has also played its part, eroding not just her body but her mind as well. It's as if both diseases are conspiring, working together to slowly dismantle Clara's essence.

She knows there is something she should remember, something deeper than names or dates. She knows that somewhere in her mind are stories, anecdotes, precious memories of happy moments, but she cannot reach them. Every time she tries to focus, it feels as if she's in a room filled with smoke, searching for a door she cannot see. The confusion is tangible. She looks at the photograph again, trying to find answers in those familiar faces, but all she feels is an immense loneliness.

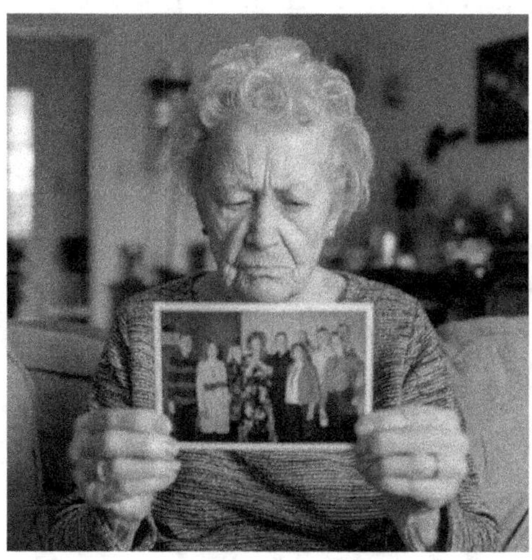

Fragments of Identity

Clara hadn't always been this way. There was a time when her mind was clear, her memory sharp as a blade. She remembered every birthday, every anniversary, every little joke she shared with her husband. She knew by heart her children's full names, their birth dates, their favorite foods. Now, those memories, once so present and accessible, have transformed into shadows, echoes of what once was.

The fragments of her identity—those moments that defined her as a wife, mother, and friend—are crumbling. How does one define a person when their memory fades? For Clara, this question is a constant struggle. She looks at the photo and knows that image is tangible proof that she was once loved and that she once loved. But she no longer has access to the stories that connected her to those faces. It's as if she's looking at a stranger's life.

In her hands, the photograph seems to weigh more than usual, not because of the wooden frame or the glass, but because of the symbolic weight it represents. Clara feels it deep in her soul, though she cannot express what's passing through her mind. It's a sense of loss that goes beyond words, a void that cannot be filled, no matter how hard she tries to hold onto the few memories she has left.

The Silence of the Mind

The silence inside her mind is deafening. Once, her head was full of thoughts, of laughter, of conversations with people who

now only exist in photographs. She could remember the sounds of her children's voices when they were small, the soft purring of her husband's car as he arrived home after a long day at work. But now, that internal noise has been replaced by a void—a void that consumes everything around it.

Clara tries to focus on the image, hoping that something, anything, will emerge from that silence. She looks into her children's eyes in the photo. She tries to remember the sound of their laughter. She knows the answer is somewhere in her mind, but it's as if it's trapped behind an invisible wall, out of reach.

Sometimes, for a few brief moments, a spark of memory seems to ignite. A fleeting flash of clarity, a sense of recognition. "This is my husband," she tells herself. "These are my daughters." But as quickly as it appears, that spark fades, leaving only darkness behind.

Alzheimer's has done its work patiently, erasing piece by piece, until she is left alone with that overwhelming void. And diabetes, with its own devastating effects, has hastened the process, eroding her ability to hold on to those fragments of identity that still defined her. What remains is a mind trapped in a constant struggle to survive in a landscape where everything familiar is vanishing.

The Spark That Persists

Despite everything, there is still something in Clara's eyes that shines—a small spark of what once was. In her most lucid moments, that spark becomes a faint flame, like a beacon trying to guide her back to reality. Sometimes, it's a smile that crosses her face for no apparent reason, as if, for a second, her mind remembers the happiness of a time long past.

It is that spark that keeps a small part of Clara alive, that part of her soul that neither Alzheimer's nor diabetes can fully extinguish. That spark is the love she once felt for the people in the photo. Even though their names and their stories have faded, the feeling remains, buried deep within her being.

It is a love that doesn't need words or detailed memories to exist. It is the love of a mother for her children, the love of a wife for her husband, the love of a woman who, though she can no longer express all that she once was, still holds within her that small spark of humanity. That spark is all that remains in a world where everything else has been lost.

The Light Fading Slowly

However, that spark, no matter how small and persistent, is in danger of going out. Each day is a new battle, a constant struggle to maintain her connection to the outside world, to avoid being completely engulfed by the darkness that surrounds her. But it's a battle Clara is losing, and she knows it, even if she can't express it in words.

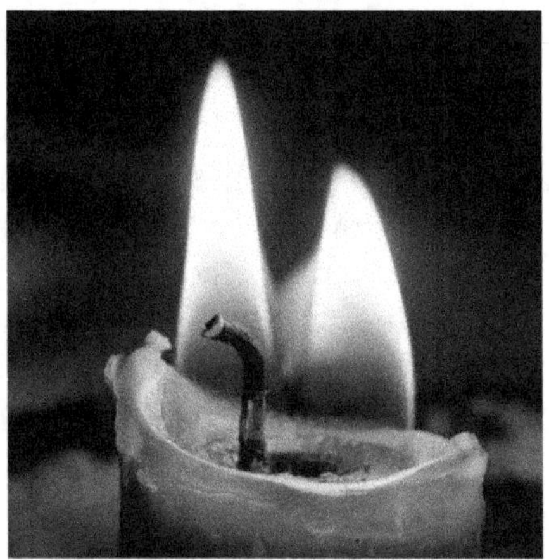

Each time she looks at the photo, that small light inside her seems to flicker, like a candle on the verge of going out. The memories that once defined her as a mother, wife, and friend are fading, leaving only shadows behind. But as long as she continues to hold that photograph, as long as her fingers caress those faces, a part of her keeps fighting, keeps resisting, clinging to what remains.

Clara knows she is at a crossroads. The empty reality she lives in is a reflection of her own mind, a place where memories have ceased to exist, where the connections that once tied her to her family and her identity have broken. But as long as that spark keeps burning, even for just one more moment, Clara is still Clara. And for now, that is enough.

Chapter 4: The Future in Our Hands

Leticia stood watching her mother, Doña Clara, who sat by the window with a distant gaze, holding the same family photo she had caressed so many times over the past few weeks. The image of her mother, a woman who had always been strong and steady, crumbled before her like a sandcastle facing the sea. She was no longer the vibrant woman who had raised her, but a fragile version of herself, trapped in a silent spiral of forgetfulness.

Alzheimer's had slowly consumed Clara, stripping away her memories, her identity, and, ultimately, her connection to the loved ones who once surrounded her. Leticia had witnessed every step of this painful process, from the first innocent lapses in memory to the moments when her mother could no longer recognize her own children. She had tried to deny it at first, seeking answers from doctors, books, even home remedies that promised to slow the inevitable. But nothing had worked. Now, all that remained was the silent pain of accepting reality.

Still, as she looked at Clara, Leticia didn't only feel sadness. There was something more—a mixture of fear and responsibility that intertwined with her grief. Tears ran down her cheeks, but her mind was elsewhere, projecting into the future, thinking about what was to come for her and her family. Leticia couldn't help but think of her own fate, of the possibility that one day she too might face the same dark destiny.

The Legacy of Alzheimer's and Diabetes

Leticia knew that Alzheimer's was not a battle fought in

isolation. The connection between Alzheimer's and diabetes had been the subject of countless nights of research and conversations with doctors. The two diseases were intertwined, like branches of the same poisoned tree. Diabetes, which had accompanied Clara for years, had not only ravaged her body but had also wreaked havoc on her mind, accelerating neural damage and undermining her brain's defenses.

It was a terrifying legacy. Leticia felt trapped between two struggles: helping her mother navigate the labyrinth of forgetfulness and protecting herself from the same fate. Genetics didn't lie. She knew the same risk of diabetes ran through her veins, and with it, a higher likelihood of cognitive decline. That realization was, in many ways, more frightening than the disease itself. It wasn't just a threat to her but to her children. This battle wasn't hers alone; it belonged to her family, to future generations.

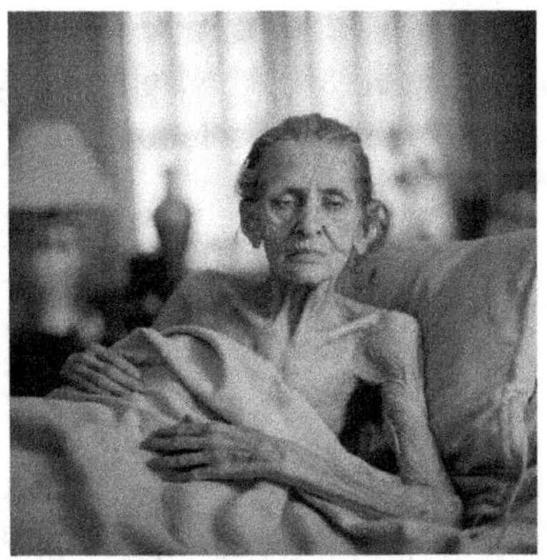

She approached her mother's bed, where Clara continued to gaze out the window. Slowly, Leticia sat beside her, taking her hand. The cold touch of Clara's skin reminded her of how much had changed. This woman, who had once been the pillar of her life, now needed more care than ever. Yet, Clara gently squeezed her daughter's hand, a small gesture that, though silent, told Leticia that, in some way, her mother was still there.

A New Resolution

Watching her mother in that state filled Leticia with an iron determination. Leticia knew she couldn't change what had happened—couldn't rewrite the past or return the memories Alzheimer had stolen from her mother. But what she *could* do was take control of the present and the future. There was a decision she had avoided for a long time, a change that now seemed not only necessary but urgent.

She needed to take care of herself, of her health. And not just for her own sake, but for her children. The battle against Alzheimer's and diabetes wasn't just a fight against forgetfulness—it was a fight for life itself, for the quality of the years she had left and for the legacy she would leave to her descendants. Leticia felt responsible not only for her own well-being but also for that of future generations. She didn't want her children to look at her one day with the same lost expression that now greeted her from her mother's eyes.

In that moment, Leticia decided she would do everything possible to slow the advance of these diseases in her own life. She knew there was no guarantee of avoiding Alzheimer's, but she also knew that prevention was her best weapon. She had learned that diabetes wasn't just a matter of sugar or insulin—

it was a disease that affected every part of the body, including the brain. And if she could prevent it or at least control it, perhaps she could protect her neurons, her memories, and, ultimately, her identity.

The First Steps Toward Change

Leticia thought about how she should approach this challenge, how to make meaningful changes in her life—not just for herself, but also for her children, who were starting to grow up and form their own habits. She knew it wasn't just about going on a diet or taking more walks. It was about a complete shift in how she lived her life. It would be a slow change, but a fundamental one.

First, she would seek medical advice. She needed to know her risk level for both diabetes and Alzheimer's. She knew that recent studies showed that controlling blood sugar could reduce the risk of cognitive decline, and she wanted to be up to date on the latest research. She would seek help from experts, but she also knew that there were things that depended on her, on her willpower to make changes.

Exercise would be key. Leticia had read that regular physical movement not only improved metabolic health but also strengthened the brain, helping to create new neural connections. She decided to start with daily walks. It was a small step, but a significant one. It wasn't just for her body— it was for her mind, for her future.

A Legacy for Her Children

Leticia glanced toward the hallway, where she could hear her children laughing in another room. She knew she also needed to teach them the importance of caring for their health. She didn't want them to carry the same fear she felt, but she did want them to understand the value of prevention. It wasn't just about longevity—it was about quality of life. It was about reaching old age with a clear mind, with the ability to remember the faces and stories that make up a person's life.

She was determined to change her family's narrative. To break the cycle of diseases that had affected her mother and now threatened to touch her as well. She knew that educating her children was essential. She would include them in her new routines, take them on walks, talk to them about the importance of healthy eating—but she would do it in a way that didn't scare them, but inspired them.

Leticia understood that the battle wasn't just against Alzheimer's and diabetes, but against the unhealthy habits that were often passed down from generation to generation without question. It was a fight against complacency, against neglect. Because the future of her family, the legacy she would leave her children, was not only measured in memories but also in the care they took of their bodies and minds.

The Future in Our Hands

As she held her mother's hand, Leticia felt a new peace, a sense of acceptance, but also an unshakable conviction. The future was in her hands. She couldn't predict it or control every aspect of it, but she could influence it. She could protect her health, her children's health, and teach them to value their physical and mental well-being.

The tears that streamed down her face were now tears of resolve. Leticia knew the fight against these diseases was bigger than herself, bigger than her mother, but she also knew that she could do her part. Prevention wasn't just about numbers or statistics—it was about love, about legacy, about protecting the people she loved most.

Clara's story, though tragic, would not be the end of their family. Leticia would do whatever it took to ensure that future generations could look back and remember—not just with love, but with clarity. Because the battle against forgetfulness isn't just an individual struggle; it's a fight for life itself. And Leticia was ready to fight with all her strength.

Chapter 5: The Dark Link Between Alzheimer's and Diabetes

Leticia had spent months researching, asking doctors, and reading every scientific article she could find. Each word she read reinforced an inescapable truth: Alzheimer's and diabetes were more connected than she had ever imagined. Her mother, Doña Clara, had lived with type 2 diabetes for years—a diagnosis that, at the time, seemed manageable with medication and diet, but was now revealing a much more sinister side, one that extended far beyond blood sugar issues.

Alzheimer's, the devastating disease that had slowly stolen Clara's memories and identity, had roots not only in genetics or aging but also in diabetes. For Leticia, understanding this connection was like discovering that the enemy that had destroyed her mother's life had been inside her long before the first symptoms of forgetfulness appeared.

Insulin Resistance in the Brain: A Brain That Forgets How to Function

One of the discoveries that impacted Leticia the most was the concept of insulin resistance in the brain. She knew that in type 2 diabetes, the body becomes less sensitive to insulin, leading to problems with regulating blood sugar. But what she hadn't understood until now was that the same process could occur in the brain. The brain cells of people with Alzheimer's, just like the cells in the body of someone with diabetes, become unable to properly process insulin—a hormone vital not only for glucose metabolism but also for the proper functioning of neurons.

In Leticia's mind, this was like turning on a light in the darkness. Insulin resistance wasn't just affecting her mother's body—it was preventing her brain from getting the energy it needed to function. It was as if Clara's brain had forgotten how to be a brain, how to switch on its circuits and keep the connections that gave coherence to her thoughts alive. Could it be that Alzheimer's, a disease she had always seen as a mysterious and tragic force, was in part the result of something as concrete as a metabolic imbalance?

Chronic Inflammation: The Silent Fire That Destroys the Brain

Inflammation was another concept Leticia had had to familiarize herself with. Type 2 diabetes generates low-grade systemic inflammation that, although painless, slowly damages the body's tissues. What she had never suspected was that this silent fire was also burning in the brain. Studies suggested that this chronic inflammation could be contributing to the neurodegeneration her mother suffered from day to day.

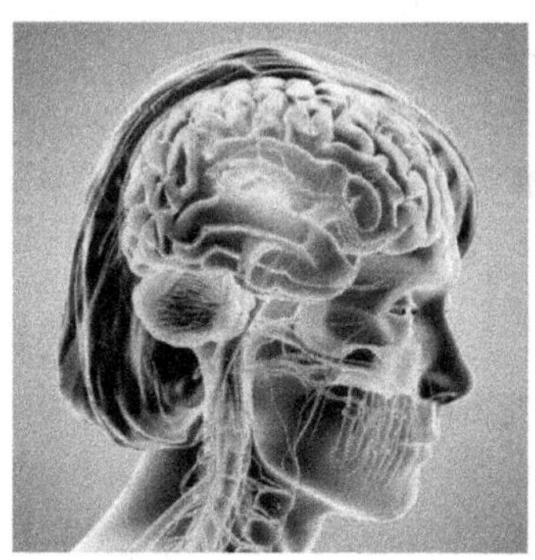

Leticia imagined her mother's brain as a vast field where small flames ignited in the deepest corners, destroying the delicate connections between neurons. Each spark of inflammation damaged her ability to remember, recognize, and think clearly. It was a desolate image, but it helped Leticia understand why things had deteriorated so quickly.

Oxidative Stress: The Relentless Wear on Cells

The concept of oxidative stress was more familiar to Leticia. She knew that diabetes was associated with the production of free radicals, molecules that damage cells and accelerate aging. But, as with inflammation, the damage wasn't confined to the body. This oxidative stress also affected the brain, speeding up cognitive decline.

For Leticia, it was as if her mother's brain had been exposed to relentless corrosion, a kind of invisible rust that gradually wore down her neuronal cells, leaving them vulnerable to damage and death. The brain, like the body, was aging prematurely, crumbling under the weight of oxidative stress.

Vascular Problems: A Heart That Doesn't Reach the Brain

Over the years, Clara had suffered from vascular complications related to diabetes—poor circulation, small wounds that took too long to heal, complaints of tired and aching legs. But Leticia had never imagined that these same problems were affecting her mother's brain in such a devastating way.

The blood vessels in the brain, just like in other parts of the body, deteriorated with diabetes. This reduced blood flow, depriving neurons of the oxygen and nutrients they needed to stay healthy. Leticia saw it clearly: her mother was not just losing her ability to remember; she was also losing the vitality that good circulation would have provided. It was as if a vital highway to her brain had been cut off, leaving the neurons isolated and doomed to die.

Beta-Amyloid Plaques: The Hidden Enemy

Perhaps the most disturbing discovery for Leticia was the presence of beta-amyloid plaques. These protein buildups, which block communication between neurons, are one of the most distinctive features of Alzheimer's. To Leticia, they had always been a kind of villain in the story of her mother's disease, but what she hadn't understood until now was how type 2 diabetes could be linked to their formation.

Studies suggested that diabetes didn't just damage the body through insulin resistance or inflammation; it could also accelerate the accumulation of these plaques in the brain. The idea that the same mechanisms causing her mother's metabolic complications might also be behind the destruction of her brain filled Leticia with a quiet anguish. The connection between Alzheimer's and diabetes was far deeper than she had ever imagined.

Prevention: A Future in Our Hands

As Leticia delved deeper into her research, she realized that

preventing Alzheimer's and diabetes wasn't just possible—it was essential. She understood that taking care of her own brain and metabolism now, while there was still time, was the best way to protect her future. She knew she couldn't change her mother's fate, but she could influence her own and that of her children.

The idea that Alzheimer's could be considered a kind of "type 3 diabetes" gave Leticia a new perspective. It was as if the pieces of a puzzle were finally starting to fit together. For her, the key lay in prevention, in taking steps to keep her blood sugar levels under control, reduce inflammation, and care for her vascular and brain health. Leticia was determined not to repeat the cycle.

Her mother's story would not be her own.

Chapter 6: The First Steps of Forgetting

Twenty years ago, Clara was a different woman. In those days, she was the unshakable pillar of her family, a figure of strength and dedication who balanced her work, home, and the countless responsibilities that came with being a mother, wife, and professional. Each day began before dawn, with the alarm clock ringing too early, yet it never slowed her pace.

Clara worked as a manager at a supply company, a position she had earned through hard work and perseverance. She was a decisive woman, known for her ability to handle multiple tasks at once. Endless phone calls, back-to-back meetings, and quick decisions were part of her daily life. The respect she had gained from her colleagues was notable. They knew they could rely on Clara to solve problems that seemed unsolvable.

At home, it was no different. Upon arriving from work, Clara transformed into a mother and wife, without pausing for a moment. She prepared dinner for her family, helped her children with their homework, and ensured that everything in the household ran smoothly. Her days seemed endless, but she did it with a smile. Fatigue wasn't something that could stop her. There was too much at stake, and her family depended on her.

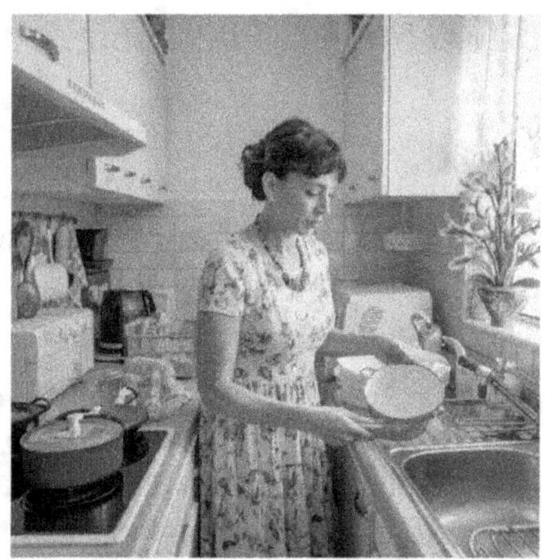

The Diagnosis: A Silenced Warning

One day, during a routine doctor's visit, Clara received news that would change her life forever, though she didn't realize it at the time. "You have type 2 diabetes," the doctor said with a tone of concern. Clara, with her phone vibrating in her bag from work messages, heard the words but didn't fully absorb them.

"Diabetes," she thought. It didn't sound that serious at the moment. She knew others lived with the disease, and in her busy mind, diabetes seemed like just another problem she could deal with later. The doctor recommended immediate lifestyle changes: a healthy diet, regular exercise, and strict control of her glucose levels. Clara nodded, took the pamphlets offered to her, and left the office.

But as soon as she crossed the door, her mind returned to the avalanche of tasks awaiting her. She had a meeting that afternoon and hadn't yet prepared the reports. Her daughter, Leticia, needed materials for a school project, and her husband had a work trip for which he needed her help organizing the details. "I'll take care of this later," she told herself. "When I have time."

The Race Against Time

Time. That was what Clara always seemed to lack. Her life was a continuous race against the clock. During those years, there seemed to be no space for anything other than work, family, and solving the day's problems. Every minute was scheduled, and every hour was assigned to a task. Diabetes, while it sounded serious, wasn't something that could stop her. It wasn't an immediate emergency.

"I'll make changes when things calm down," she promised herself. But that day never came. There was always something more urgent, always another important meeting or a problem that couldn't wait. Often, she skipped meals or ate whatever was on her desk—cookies, chips, anything that could fill her up quickly so she could keep going. Exercise simply didn't fit into her schedule. There was no time to walk or go to the gym, let alone cook healthy meals every day.

In the first few months after the diagnosis, Clara tried to follow some of the doctor's recommendations. She bought fresh vegetables and a stationary bike that, after a few weeks, began collecting dust in a corner of the house. "It's not the right time," she told herself. "When things settle down, I'll focus on my health." But things never settled down.

The First Symptoms: A Warning Ignored

Over time, Clara began noticing small changes in her body, but she attributed them to stress and fatigue. She felt more tired than usual, but who wouldn't with so much on their mind? Sometimes she felt dizzy or noticed her vision was a bit blurry. "It's from spending too many hours in front of the computer," she told herself, convincing herself there was nothing to worry about.

The weight gain was another symptom she couldn't entirely ignore, but she chalked it up to getting older. "It's normal," she thought. "After 40, metabolism changes." Although she knew deep down that her diet and lack of exercise were contributing factors, there simply wasn't time to do anything about it.

As diabetes silently progressed, Clara began experiencing more memory problems—small lapses that at first seemed trivial. She forgot names in meetings, details of important conversations, and sometimes even the tasks she had assigned to her team. She told herself it was just fatigue, the stress of trying to do everything. After all, she was still efficient at her job, though it took more effort.

The doctor continued to warn her at every visit: "Clara, you need to take this disease seriously." But she kept postponing the recommendations. Sometimes she took her prescribed pills, but other times she forgot or delayed them. "I have so much on my mind," she thought. Her family also reminded her of the importance of taking care of herself, but she always responded with the same phrase: "I'm fine, everything's under control."

The Cost of Neglected Self-Care

What Clara didn't see, or perhaps couldn't or didn't want to admit, was that diabetes doesn't wait. It is a silent disease that attacks from within, without making noise, until the damage is irreversible. And while Clara kept putting off her self-care, the disease progressed.

Years passed, and Clara remained submerged in her frantic life, increasingly trapped in the endless cycle of obligations. She didn't notice that her forgetfulness was becoming more frequent or that her energy was waning. Her body was trying to send her signals, but she didn't have time to listen. Each year that passed without paying attention to her health, without adjusting her diet or incorporating exercise, was paving the way for deterioration.

It was ironic, Leticia thought years later, to see how such a strong and capable woman had fallen victim to a disease that, with a bit of attention, could have been managed. Clara had dedicated her life to caring for her family and her work, but had never reserved time to care for herself.

The Beginning of the Decline

Clara's decline wasn't sudden. It was a gradual process, starting with small symptoms that seemed insignificant but, by ignoring them, grew until they became uncontrollable. The memory problems turned into confusion. The brief lapses became moments of total disconnection. When Clara finally began to notice that something deeper was wrong, it was already too late.

Diabetes, that silent enemy, had paved the way for something much more devastating: Alzheimer's. Her body, weakened by years of poor health management, could no longer defend itself. The connections in her brain that had once defined her as a capable and strong woman began to crumble, just as her ability to keep her blood sugar under control had.

Now, two decades later, Clara could barely remember who she was. But Leticia remembered. She remembered the tireless mother, the strong woman who had sacrificed so much for her family. And now, seeing what had happened, Leticia promised herself that she would not repeat the same mistakes.

Chapter 7: The Cost of Caring

Leticia was exhausted. She felt it in her bones, in the heaviness of her eyelids, and in the slow rhythm of her thoughts. The day began as it always did, with the sound of the alarm reminding her of the endless list of tasks she had to complete. But this list wasn't filled with work responsibilities or personal projects. It was a list dedicated to Clara, her mother, who now depended on her for almost everything.

Since Alzheimer's had progressed, Leticia's life had completely transformed. Her days were organized around caring for her mother, and that had started to consume every part of her being. At first, it was something she accepted naturally. After all, it was her mother. Who better than her to care for her during these moments? But over time, that acceptance had turned into a silent burden that was slowly but surely wearing her down.

The daily routine was predictable, yet exhausting. Every morning, Leticia made sure her mother got up, took her medications, and ate something nutritious, though Clara often refused or couldn't understand what she needed to do. Some days, her mother was irritable, and on others, she simply sat in silence, staring blankly. Leticia tried to fill those silences, searching for something, anything, to bring her mother back, even if only for a brief moment.

Involuntary Isolation

What Leticia hadn't foreseen was how this caregiving role was isolating her from her own life. Her friends had stopped calling as often. At first, she declined invitations to go out, explaining that she had too many responsibilities at home. "Maybe another time," she would say, but that "another time" never came. Eventually, the invitations stopped coming. Now, her phone hardly rang, and when it did, it was for reminders of doctor's appointments or calls from the pharmacy.

Her husband, Miguel, tried to be understanding, but Leticia could see that he was tired too. Their conversations had become brief, almost transactional, limited to discussing who would pick up the kids or what groceries to buy. They no longer talked about their dreams, their worries, or simply how their day had been. The spark that once connected them was fading, and Leticia didn't know how to reignite it. The house felt smaller, as if every corner was saturated with the weight of constant caregiving.

The most painful thing, however, was the time spent with her children. Leticia had once been an active mother, involved in all her kids' activities. But now, her energy was drained. The nights they used to spend reading together had turned into nights when Leticia, exhausted, fell asleep on the couch. Her eldest son, Lucas, had stopped asking her for help with his homework, knowing that her mind was elsewhere. And the worst part was the guilt she felt for not being there for them, knowing that they needed her too.

The Invisible Burden of Caregiving

What few people saw, what almost no one understood, was the emotional toll that came with caring for someone who was no longer the person you once knew. Leticia loved her mother; she always had. But now, Clara was no longer the strong and determined woman who had raised her. Now, she was someone different, someone who needed constant care and, in her most difficult moments, didn't even recognize her own daughter.

There were days when Leticia was overwhelmed by a sadness she couldn't express. A part of her knew she was losing her mother, but another part resisted accepting that reality. Alzheimer's hadn't just stolen Clara's memories; it had also stolen Leticia's relationship with her mother. Each time Clara looked at her with those empty eyes, asking if she was the nurse, Leticia felt a piece of herself break.

She had tried to be strong. She had tried not to show her emotions in front of her mother, but over time, those emotions had begun to accumulate like a weight on her chest. Leticia had put her own life, her own dreams, on hold to care for her mother, and though she never regretted that decision, she couldn't help but feel trapped.

Caregiver Syndrome: A Silent Burnout

She had heard of caregiver syndrome, but she never thought it would happen to her. At first, she didn't notice the symptoms. The persistent headaches, the insomnia that kept her awake in the middle of the night, the moments when she felt on the verge of tears for no apparent reason—all seemed like normal consequences of exhaustion. But then other signs began to appear.

Leticia started to feel easily frustrated. Small things, like when Clara refused to eat or when she didn't remember who Leticia was, began to make her lose her patience. She felt guilty for feeling that way. "It's not her fault," she repeated to herself, but that didn't make the frustration go away. She also began to experience a sense of hopelessness. There were moments when she wondered if things would ever get better, if there would be an end to this endless cycle of caregiving.

It was during one of the few times she allowed herself to cry in solitude that Leticia realized something had to change. She couldn't go on like this. Not only was she losing her mother, but she was losing herself. She couldn't keep ignoring her own well-being. She knew that if she continued this way, eventually, she wouldn't have the energy to care for anyone— not her mother, not her family, not even herself.

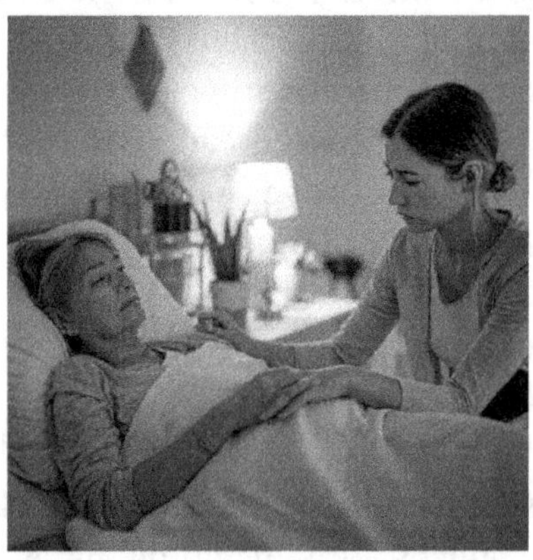

The Need for Support

One day, during a conversation with a friend who had gone through a similar experience, Leticia realized something fundamental: she didn't have to do it all alone. There were people, support networks, and professionals who could help her bear the burden. "Asking for help isn't a sign of weakness," her friend said, "it's what will allow you to keep going."

Leticia decided to seek help. She reached out to a caregiver support group where others shared their experiences and challenges. It wasn't easy to open up, but hearing others' stories made her feel less alone. There was something comforting in knowing she wasn't the only one who felt that way—that her exhaustion and frustration were valid.

She also sought professional help for her mother's care. She couldn't do everything, and that was okay. She found a caregiver to assist during the day, which allowed her to reclaim some of her time and energy. Little by little, Leticia began to feel like she could breathe again.

Self-Care: An Act of Self-Love

As she stopped carrying the entire weight of caregiving alone, Leticia began to remember something she had forgotten: her own self-care. She started making small changes, like taking morning walks, setting aside a few minutes to meditate, and reconnecting with her own thoughts. She also began spending more time with her children, recovering those lost moments she had missed so much.

She understood that caring for her mother didn't mean

abandoning her own life. In fact, taking care of herself was a way to honor Clara, ensuring she had the energy and love to give her mother the best of herself. Leticia learned that in order to care for others, she first had to care for herself.

And so, while Alzheimer's continued its course in her mother's life, Leticia found a new way to live with the disease. She was no longer alone in the battle, and that gave her the strength to move forward, not just for Clara, but also for herself.

Chapter 8: Conversations with the Past

Leticia sat in the dim light of her room, perched on the edge of the bed with her hands clasped and her elbows resting on her knees. The house was silent, a rare occurrence in recent times, but exhaustion had finally caught up to her, and she had managed to get her mother, Clara, to sleep deeply after a long day full of repetitions and forgetfulness.

That night, however, Leticia couldn't sleep. The weight of the past few years seemed to press down on her chest, a burden not only from the present but also from the past. She closed her eyes, searching for a moment of peace, but instead, a flood of thoughts began to invade her mind, taking her to places she hadn't visited in a long time.

What would have happened if everything had been different? If she had known what the future held for them? If she had done something earlier? It was a conversation she had often had in silence with herself, but this time it was different. This time, it felt as if her past self was standing right in front of her, waiting for an answer. And in that moment, Leticia decided to confront the conversation she had avoided for so long.

"If I Had Known..."

"If I had known what I know now," Leticia whispered softly, as if speaking to a younger version of herself. She imagined sitting across from that woman from twenty years ago, the Leticia who still saw her mother as an unbreakable force, a woman capable of facing the world and winning. That Leticia had yet to understand that time and illness could change people, much less that her mother would come to depend on her in such a painful way.

"If I had known what was coming," Leticia continued, "I would have done everything I could to take better care of you, Mom." Her words were a whisper, as if speaking to the wind. But in her mind, she was addressing both her mother and that younger version of herself, the one who still had the chance to change things.

"I would have insisted that you take diabetes more seriously. I wouldn't have let you ignore the doctor's warnings. I would have learned more about the disease myself, done research, gone with you to every doctor's appointment. Because now I know what I didn't know then: that diabetes wasn't just a blood sugar problem. It was something much bigger, something that was waiting to tear us apart."

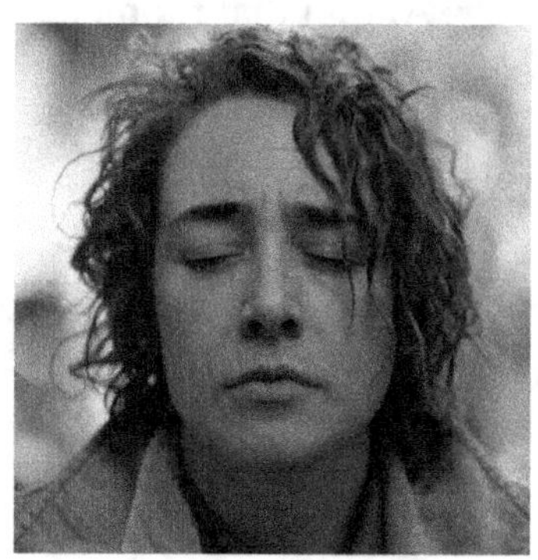

Leticia closed her eyes tightly, trying to hold back the tears that were beginning to form. "I would have done more. I would have convinced you that you couldn't keep going as if nothing was wrong. I would have cooked healthier meals, walked with you every day, pushed you to move, to take care of yourself. I would have insisted, Mom. I would have been firmer, more attentive…"

"I'm Sorry for Not Doing More"

The tears finally spilled over, running hot and bitter down her cheeks. "I'm sorry for not doing more when I still could. For not giving you the importance you deserved when Alzheimer's and diabetes could still have been slowed. For not caring for you the way you cared for me. I'm sorry for not realizing that this disease was taking more from you than I could see."

The pain she had been suppressing for so long finally rose to the surface. She felt the weight of regret, of missed opportunities, of days when she had been too busy with her own life, her own problems, without realizing that her mother had been fighting a silent battle against a disease that would end up consuming them both.

"If I could go back, Mom, I would have made you understand that you weren't alone, that I was there to help you, but that you needed to help me help you. I would have talked to you more about the importance of your health, would have done whatever it took to make you take every warning, every symptom, seriously."

Leticia took a deep breath, and in the dark silence of the night, she felt as though she was not only connecting with her mother but also with all the decisions she had made over the years. But something else emerged from that pain: a kind of clarity, an understanding.

"This Isn't Just a Warning, It's a Call"

As she opened her eyes, Leticia realized that she was no longer just speaking to her past. She understood that this dialogue wasn't only for herself, or just for her mother. It was a message that, somehow, she needed to share. It was advice that, through her own experience, had become an undeniable truth.

"If you're reading this," Leticia whispered, imagining her words might reach someone else, "if you ever find yourself in the same situation I was in, take care of the ones you love before it's too late. Don't ignore the warning signs. Don't expect time to heal everything. Time, on its own, is not enough. Learn about the disease. Talk about it. Don't be afraid to insist, even if it means being uncomfortable or seeming pushy. Because believe me, a difficult conversation today can save you so much tomorrow."

The tears stopped, but Leticia still felt the deep sadness that came with the realization. However, that sadness also began to transform into honest advice, into a warning she wished she had received years ago.

"Talk to your family. Learn to listen to the silences. Don't let the routine distance you from what truly matters. Because a disease like Alzheimer's or diabetes doesn't show its true face until it's too late. But if you act now, if you make the effort to prevent what can be prevented, to care for what is still in your hands… then maybe you can avoid the pain I now carry."

A Different Future

Leticia sat in silence for several minutes, her mind finally calming. She realized that although she couldn't change the past, she could still influence the future. She could still take care of her own health, of her family, and of the people who still had time to learn from her experience.

"It's not too late for others," she thought, feeling a slight hope emerge from her sadness. "I can't change what happened with my mother, but if my words reach someone who still has time, then maybe this story won't just be one of pain, but also of prevention, of change."

Leticia understood that this internal conversation, this grieving with the past, had been necessary—not to relive the guilt, but to free herself from it. Her mother could no longer become the woman she once was, but perhaps others could still avoid the same fate.

And with that understanding, Leticia allowed herself, for the first time in a long while, to rest. She had done what she could, and now her mission was to share the message that her experience had taught her. Because, in the end, preventing future harm was the greatest act of love she could offer—not only to her mother but also to those who still had time.